Fecal Transplant

Early History of FMT

Yashi Nozawa

Yashi Nozawa

ISBN-13: 978-1507834633

ISBN-10: 1507834632

Published by ITP in partnership with
CreateSpace

Indian Town Press (ITP)

P.O.Box 1764

Indiantown, FL 34956

Dedication

To my wife, Ann W. Nozawa

For her love, assistance and support

Table of Contents

Chapter 1: A Pretty Lady

Betty is probably the prettiest lady in our mobile park, in which all residents are retired persons. It is a typical Florida "fifty-five plus" resident community. People who live here are free-spirited, and they do anything their hearts desire. She is a naturally aging attractive lady and probably over sixty years old. I had noticed her for a while and was looking for an opportunity to become acquainted with her. So far, I never had the chance. One day she stopped me while I was riding my bicycle as my daily exercise.

"Hi, we never met, but I believe you are Yashi, who writes short stories in our monthly community newsletters."

"Yes I am the one. Well, nice to meet you ma'am. What can I do for you?"

"Don't be formal with me like that. I am Betty. Please call me Betty."

"OKay. What can I do for you, Betty?"

"I want to talk to you privately. Can we set a time? Any time that's convenient for you. Probably it

will take one or at most two hours in my house here."
She pointed out the house behind her.

I was excited and wondered what she wanted to
talk about. Anyway, I was glad to have a chance to talk
with a pretty lady about whatever the subject would be,
especially in private conversation.

"How about tomorrow afternoon after lunch, say
two o'clock?" I said.

On the next day, I visited her at the appointed
time. She invited me into her house. The inside was
well kept and decorated modestly in good taste.
Marvelous pictures were on the walls and knickknacks
were placed here and there at strategic places. I could
not figure out her background or her interests from
these items. The only idea I could get was that she was
living alone, like many other ladies in this community.

She pointed out a seat by a round glass-top table,
"Please sit down. What kind of drink would you like to
have?"

"Some kind of a soft drink is OK. If you have a
diet one, I prefer it. If you don't have it, any non-
alcoholic drink will do the job."

She brought two glasses of diet Coke with ice
and placed them on the table. I was eager to hear her
story, but she seemed not ready to start. We chatted a
while. Eventually, I became impatient and said, "Betty,
I feel you may regret that you have decided to talk with
me. So, if you are not ready I will come back some

other time, or if you want, we can cancel the whole plan without any qualms."

"I am sorry. It is really hard for me, but I have to talk with you now. Otherwise, we may never have another chance. Excuse me, just a second." She stood up and brought back a newspaper.

"Did you read this paper?" It was a recent issue of *The Palm Beach Post*, a local paper.

"Yes, I subscribe to the paper, so I probably read whatever the story was, because I usually read the paper through from beginning to end."

The article she pointed out was *Nightmare Bacteria: Antibiotic-resistant Germs in Florida*, the headline article in the June 22, 2014 Sunday edition. I nodded without saying anything.

"Then, you read this article too." She flipped several sheets and showed an article titled, *Transplant with an 'Ick' Factor Has Amazing Results*.

I almost opened my mouth and was ready to say, "You were one of the...," but I kept silent and just nodded.

"I was ashamed and traumatized by incessant peer teasing. I kept the incident secret for a long time. But when I read the article, I decided that I had to tell my story for the sake of history."

The following amazing true story was based on Betty's confession. However, because of her wishes, I changed all names and places, including Betty's name, in order to avoid any potential legal complications.

Sixty years ago, Betty was a nursing student in a world-renowned research hospital, Universal Benevolent General Hospital (UBG) in a Western country. In her senior year, she had a patient called Mr. Patterson.

He was originally hospitalized for stomach surgery. The surgery was successful, but he developed complications during his post-operative recovery phase. He suffered from a high fever and severe diarrhea. Doctors treated him with antibiotics, but his condition was worsening almost every day. His problem was diagnosed as pseudo-membranous colitis (PM colitis), which had no known cure.

He was very sick and wasting away every day. Doctors had tried everything they knew. He seemed to have a digestive problem. He could not eat or drink and had severe diarrhea constantly. Doctors tried all known antibiotics and anti-diarrhea medicines without any effect. The patient was suffering extreme dehydration and malnutrition. He seemed to have no more muscles or fat left on his body; he was all skin and bones. He already looked like a corpse from a Nazi concentration camp. He was still conscious, but too weak to speak. Intravenous (IV) feeding could not keep up with his steady weight loss. He was ready to die at any moment.

One day when several doctors gathered to discuss what they could do about Mr. Patterson, they agreed that he would die soon unless they could find some new treatments or medications for him. Several minutes passed without any comments from anybody. Then the chief of the resident doctors faced a nearby group of nursing students nervously watching the doctor's group. He jokingly said, "Hey, student nurses, do you have any good suggestion?" He simply wanted to change the mood of the doctors. Surprisingly to the chief, one nursing student raised her hand.

"OK, let's hear it."

"Did you try yellow dragon soup?"

"Ha? What is yellow dragon soup?"

"I heard this from my Chinese friend. According to her, yellow dragon soup has a miracle power to cure the most severe diarrhea. Her grandfather was a traditional Chinese medicine doctor, and he told her the story."

"So what is yellow dragon soup? Do you know the recipe?"

"Yes and no."

"Spit it out now! This is a life or death emergency! What is it?"

"Well. I know, but I don't believe it."

"I don't care if you believe it or not! What is it?"

"Take a healthy person's stool and mix it with warm water. It is yellow dragon soup. The patient has to drink the soup. However, the patient must not be told its ingredients."

"Ridiculous! Old wive's tale!" one of the doctors said.

But the chief said, "Wait a minute. Even an old wive's tale often contains some truth. Let's think about it. The yellow dragon soup might be supplying a group of healthy and necessary bacteria for digestion to the patient who lost these bacteria. Of course, we cannot feed human stool to a patient, but we could supply them from the bottom end. That's it. I got an idea."

He faced the student nurse and said, "What is your name?"

"I am Betty, sir."

"Betty, you are a senior, aren't you?"

"Yes, sir."

"So you already know the procedure of giving enemas, don't you?"

"Yes sir. I already performed it on several patients."

"Good. I will give you the great honor and responsibility of performing the world's first stool transplant. Give an enema of yellow dragon soup to Mr. Patterson. Wait. The name of yellow dragon soup is too attention getting. How about calling it type B. That's it. Betty, you should give Mr. Patterson a type B enema as soon as possible."

Thus, Betty's nightmare started.

Chapter 2:

Yellow Dragon Soup

At first, Betty felt greatly honored that the doctor chose her for the task. Simultaneously, she was concerned about her responsibility. If she botched the task, the patient might die immediately after her enema. She tried hard to deny the worrisome idea. She convinced herself that it was her responsibility to perform such a procedure correctly and diligently; then nature would take care of itself. The outcome would not be her responsibility, but the patient's vitality would decide it. She would just concentrate on how to do the job without a mistake.

The immediate issue was how to find a suitable donor or donors. Even for a regular organ transplant, the finding of a matching donor is not an easy task. In her case, the donating item was not an ordinary item. It was an item that everybody would like to avoid mentioning. She could collect it secretly without the knowledge of the donor. For instance, she could gather it from a bedpan before she emptied it. Since a patient in a hospital was not a healthy person, this method was unacceptable. It was too bad. People dumped tons of feces every day, but she could not pick a couple of ounces from them.

Candidates for donors seemed to be limited to doctors or nurses, who were not particularly repelled by talking about stool or such. She pondered a while. The easiest way to solve the problem was to produce the required sample by herself. She would definitely try, but she knew that her daily habit dictated her timing. She usually moved her bowels the first thing in the early morning. When she was ordered to perform the procedure, it was near noon, and it seemed to be too late. She could wait until the next morning, but it would seem she was ducking her responsibility. As the doctors said, it was an emergency, and the patient might die at any moment. There was no time to waste! She made up her mind.

"Hi Cathy, you know what jam I am in, don't you?" She asked one of her nursing students.

"Yes, everybody knows that you have to do a poop transplant."

"Would you do me a favor? Could you produce a stool sample for me?"

"Why don't you try by yourself?"

'Of course, I will, but I usually do that in the morning, so I will not likely succeed soon. I need the sample as soon as possible, at the latest, by three o'clock this afternoon. Please could you try?"

"OK, Betty for friendship's sake, I will try."

Betty asked three more fellow students, and two agreed to try. The third student refused, saying that she had diarrhea herself.

After Betty had secured three potential donors, counting herself, she went to the cafeteria for lunch. She wondered what food she should eat to produce her sample in time. She decided her favorite food, pork chop, a double serving with plenty of drink to lubricate it. She did not enjoy the meal. She felt like she was eating as a medical test.

When she was ready to leave the cafeteria, Doctor Smith, one of the kind doctors, stopped her.

"You are Betty, aren't you?"

"Yes sir,"

"I believe you need a stool, don't you?"

"Yes, sir"

"Do you already have it?"

"No sir. I have been trying to get it, but do not yet have it, sir."

"Then, why don't you wait, say, ten minutes. I will send a sample to the collection place. So you can pick it up."

"Thank you, sir. That will be a great help. Again thank you, sir."

Betty was relieved from the tension to secure the sample. Once she relaxed, she felt like she had to go to the bathroom.

A half hour later, she went to the collection place to pick up her samples.

A lab technician asked, "So you are Betty. I wondered who was collecting so many shit samples. What are you trying to do? Are you making soup or something with them?"

"No Miss, I am trying to make type B enema fluid."

"Whatever you are trying to do, don't spill it! As you know, it stinks."

Betty had a total of four samples, including one from herself. She inspected the samples and found they all seemed to be normal looking. That caused a new problem. Which one would she use for an enema? Since she did not know how many times she would have to give a type B enema, she decided to save all of them in the freezer, except one.

If the enema were a success and the patient recovered, whose sample she used would not make too much difference. But if the patient died because of the enema, the provider of the sample might be in hot water. Betty decided to use her own. Since there was no recipe available for the enema fluid, she had to figure it out. She already decided to use a rectal bulb syringe, rather than a nozzle-bag combination, selecting a small quantity enema. Each bulb syringe could contain eight ounces, so she chose to make a total of twenty ounces allowing for an extra injection if the first attempt failed. She poured about two cups of distilled water into a beaker and put it into a bucketful of hot water to warm the beaker. When the distilled water became lukewarm, Betty removed the beaker from the hot water bath and placed it on the table. She thought this was the moment of truth.

She opened the lid of a stool sample container with her name on it. It was a stinky brown sausage. She had never carefully observed her own or anyone else's stool. She used a wooden tongue depressor to separate a half-inch long piece of the sample and dropped it into the beaker. Using the same tongue depressor, she stirred the beaker and made sure the whole sample melted. The result was a soup of brownish liquid with many small particles of solid. Luckily these particles were suspended in the water and not precipitated at the bottom. She momentarily wondered whether she should filter them or not. She decided against the filtering because these particles might be a cluster of useful bacteria. She transferred the brown soup into a bottle and put on a tight cap. When she labeled the bottle "Type B enema fluid," she suddenly questioned the wisdom of the ancient Chinese medicine man, *why did he call it Yellow Dragon Soup? It should have been named Brown Dragon Soup.* Betty tried to remember that she should ask the question when she would see her Chinese friend next time. She also placed the remaining sample into the freezer for future use.

Betty and her classmate pushed a wagon loaded with the enema supplies and other necessary items to Mr. Patterson's room. It was the scheduled time to replace his bedding. As expected, he heavily soiled his bedding. Betty's group expertly replaced the old bedding with a new sheet and a plastic protector without too much discomfort to the patient. He was aware of what was going on, but he did not say anything.

"Mr. Patterson, we will administer a new medication through your rectum using an enema device. But it is not an enema, so you should try to hold the liquid as long as possible. If you feel any pain, let me know. Are you OK?" Betty remarked. She was not sure whether he replied or not. Since he was so weak she did not expect any clear answer. So she proceeded with her procedure anyway.

She injected eight ounces of type B enema fluid into the rectum of Mr. Patterson without any mishap. She stayed there about five minutes after finishing the enema and carefully observed the patient's reactions. He seemed to be as usual; he was just lying there with closed eyes. Eventually, she left the room. She dropped into Mr. Patterson's room from time to time while she was in the area, but she could not see any change in his condition.

Chapter 3: Poop-Nurse

The next morning Betty was assigned to the same floor as Mr. Patterson. She checked the notes from the night shift and found that the nurses needed to change Mr. Patterson's soiled bedding only once, instead of every two hours. After the doctors' morning inspection of patients, the chief resident called Betty.

"Betty, congratulations, Mr. Patterson is improving. The enema of type B is working. If he deteriorates, give a booster enema. Otherwise, we keep observing his condition. Do you have any more type B enema fluid?"

"Yes sir, one more dose in a refrigerator and raw materials for additional dosages in a freezer."

"Good, keep them until further notice."

Mr. Patterson was gaining his strength at amazing speed. Next day he requested a drink and drank four ounces of apple juice. The following day he wanted to eat something. Within a couple of weeks, he was discharged from the hospital.

Unlike Mr. Patterson's recovery, Betty's condition rapidly worsened. It started with Dr. Smith.

"Hi Betty, congratulations, I am so glad to have contributed to the development of the new procedure."

Betty was annoyed and had no idea how to answer his comment. He apparently assumed that Betty used his sample for the type B enema fluid.

"Thank you, Dr. Smith. It was a great help. Excuse me. I have to see a patient who is calling." She left Dr. Smith quickly and walked toward the room of an imaginary patient.

On the same day, as soon as Cathy saw Betty, she said.

"Hi Betty, my poop worked! I am so glad I contributed to the development of a new procedure."

Betty momentarily hesitated to reply to her.

"You did use my sample, didn't you?" Cathy asked.

"Yes, of course, I used your sample. Thank you, Cathy. It was a great help."

Doris, who was another sample donor, gave Betty similar trouble. Betty had now trapped herself with her own lies because she did not have courage to tell the truth from the beginning.

Patterson's remarkable recovery became a small sensation in the Hospital. A reporter from the in-house weekly newspaper, *UBH News,* interviewed Betty. During their conversation, the subject of a donor came up.

Reporter: Who was the donor of the stool?

Betty agonized about how to answer the question.

Betty: You know, the donor might be embarrassed if I reveal the name. So, I don't want to disclose it until I get permission from them.

Reporter: You said, "them," so is there more than one donor?

Betty thought that she again dug her own grave.

Betty: Yes.

Reporter: Are they from this Hospital?

Betty: Yes.

Reporter: From staff or patients?

Betty: Of course, from staff. The donor must be a healthy person.

Reporter: Anyone from doctors?

Betty: Yes.

Reporter: Anyone from nursing staff?

Betty: Yes.

Reporter: How many in total?

Betty: Three, no, four.

Reporter: Did they include you?

Betty: Why do you think that?

Reporter: Because you forgot to count yourself at first, and then corrected.

Betty: Yes, I was one of them.

Reporter: There was a total of four donors. Did you use all of them or only one of them?

Betty had to make a choice: one or all. *If she said one, this reporter would try to find out who. The safest answer would be all.*

Betty: I used all. I mixed them, because I could not choose which one was better than others.

Reporter: Don't worry I will not ask you or seek other donors' names. Their names will be safe.

When the news of a revolutionary medical procedure to cure a difficult digestive disease appeared in the next issue of *UBH News*, Betty's problem was expanded further. The article said that a nursing student (Betty) and three other medical staff of the hospital were donors of the materials for type B enema. Betty's name spread throughout the hospital, and she got the nickname of Poop-nurse. Discussion about Poop-nurse became a favorite subject in the doctors' lounge, nursing stations, and a cafeteria. They focussed their discussion on an unexpected aspect of the incident, completely opposite of the intention of the article. The article was supposed to be praising Betty's action, but the readers' reaction was that Betty was a selfish, egocentric nurse who monopolized the glory of the new medical procedure.

Some doctors, who were new in the hospital often said to Betty with a straight face,

"So, you are the famous Poop-nurse, Betty."

Furthermore, Betty was avoided by fellow student nurses. Some of them pinched their noses when Betty approached them. The subtle gesture of a sniffing nose hurt Betty more, because it was unnoticeable to other people who did not know the background story. Therefore, student nurses used it anywhere and anytime without restriction.

Since the use of all four samples for the type B procedure became a universally accepted fact, Betty's worry increased. She eventually became paranoid about the stool sample issue. She expected that the chief resident would want to write a scientific paper and to publish it in a reputable journal. During the process, a formal bacteriological analysis would be performed. Then, the analysis might reveal that actual type B enema fluid came from a single sample. Betty decided to dispose of the type B enema fluid a few days after the appearance of the *UBH News* article, in order to protect her reputation.

Betty's daily life was already uncomfortable. She could see almost everybody displayed the sniffing motion as soon as they saw her. Every doctor seemed to be calling her Poop-nurse. She thought that if the facts about stool samples were found out, her life would become a real hell. She wondered whether the disposal of the type B enema fluid might not be enough to conceal the fact. If they checked frozen samples, they would find only one sample was not a natural sausage shape. It also would reveal the truth. So she made a big decision to dispose of all frozen samples and carried out the decision.

As she had anticipated, a few days after her disposal of all samples, the chief resident called her.

"Hi Betty, nice to see you again. I hope everything is OK with you."

"No sir, my life is hell."

"Oh, how come?"

"Everybody calls me Poop-nurse."

"Oh, that! Don't worry about it, people will forget the incident soon. By the way, I want to write a paper about type B enema. Can you bring me all remaining samples?"

"No, I cannot do it sir."

"What happened?"

"I disposed of them because they became too old and started fermenting."

"Then bring me the frozen ones."

"No, I cannot do that, either sir."

"Why?"

"Because the lab people complained about freezer space, I had to dispose of all my samples."

"Do you know what you did? The disposal of valuable medical samples without a doctor's authorization is a violation of hospital rules. You will be punished for your action. That's all."

Chapter 4: Torture Chamber

Betty was worried because she did not know what kind of punishment she might receive. Would she be expelled from the Hospital? It would mean that they might jeopardize her nursing education. Would she be suspended for a week or a month? She might not be able to endure such a punishment because her nursing education was her lifeline for her future.

A nursing instructor, Miss Hall, who had been friendly to Betty, noticed Betty's depression and asked her.

"What is going on, Betty? I noticed you seem to be unhappy."

"The chief resident said that he would punish me because I disposed of all samples of the type B enema against his orders."

"Don't worry. He was just bluffing because he was momentarily frustrated. This hospital is a huge, complicated organization. People are constantly losing or misplacing many medicines, samples, reports, etc., supposed to be irreplaceable items. If they punished every person who lost a medical sample, there would be no working staff left. If you are worried about the situation, I will find out what is going on."

"Thank you, Miss Hall, I would appreciate it if you do that."

A few days later, Miss Hall told Betty that there would be no punishment because there was no violation of Hospital rules. Betty stored the samples under her name, not with a doctor's name. So, Betty could do anything she wanted about those samples. Betty was relieved after the news. Nevertheless, her environment did not seem to have improved. Some doctors and other hospital staff still treated her with remoteness.

After a few more months in the torture chamber, Betty graduated, passed the state licensing board exam, and became a full-fledged registered nurse. Most graduate nurses went back to their home states and sought employment as staff nurses in a local hospital. Betty's hometown was the same place as Universal Benevolent General, so naturally she expected to receive an offer from them, because the hospital suffered a chronic shortage of nursing staff. However, for whatever reason, she did not receive any job offer. Of course, she could find a nursing position in another local hospital. But it would place her in an awkward position. People would wonder why she did not get a Job in UBG where she graduated. It would probably affect not only the immediate situation but also her long term career.

A lucky break came from Miss Hall, who had been watching Betty with motherly concern. She found Betty a position as an assistant instructor in the UBG nursing school. The position was as a classroom instructor with no clinical assignment. Betty would never need to step on the hospital floors where she might face her old nemesis of doctors and other medical staff.

Even though the pay of an assistant instructor was lower than that of staff nurses, she took the job and stayed about two years in that position. Meanwhile, she continued her education and acquired B.S. and M.S. degrees in Nursing Science from a local university. Then she moved to another local baccalaureate nursing school and became a professor of clinical care.

In the same period, she got married and raised three children, but she still wanted to go back to the position of a floor nurse who would engage in patient care. Once all her children were old enough to go to school, she did go back to the position of a staff nurse. The ghost of the "poop nurse" still remained in her mind, so she selected mostly night shift positions. The night shift also had the advantage: it paid better than the day shift, and she could engage with her children in afternoons after school hours. She could sleep in the mornings while the children were in school and any time she found a quiet time.

She lived relatively quietly and enjoyed a suburban middle class life for a while. A few years after all her children had left home in pursuit of their independent lives, she received an invitation for the twenty-fifth reunion from the UBG nursing school. Because of her bitter memory there, she had never attended any past reunions. Partially due to the boredom of the empty nest, she decided to attend this reunion.

They held a meeting in a plush ballroom of a five-star hotel near the hospital. When she walked into the ballroom, she was astonished. There were food kiosks, which offered various national dishes from around the world in addition to the traditional buffet tables. She also noticed that almost half the people were already drunk. Soon she found out why: there were several free bars at strategic locations in the ballroom. When she looked for former close friends, she realized that she could not identify most of the attendees. She eventually recognized a group congregated in a corner of the room.

"Hi Betty. Nice to see you! How have you been? We haven't heard from you for a long time."

"I was busy raising my kids. Now I am free so I thought it might be time to renew old friendships."

She was enjoying conversations with old friends when an unfamiliar lady approached Betty's group. She wore lots of expensive jewelry, like a walking show window of a jewel shop. She sniffed her nose and said.

"Betty! Welcome to the twenty-fifth reunion. I know you are here because I smelled it. I believe you are still in the poop business, aren't you?"

"Excuse me, who are you? I am sorry to say I cannot recognize you."

"I am Mrs. Cooney, the wife of the dot-com billionaire, John Cooney. I was the former Gabrielle Sullivan. I know you are slow, but you should recognize me. You may not know, but I am paying all the costs of today's event. So, enjoy yourself Betty, but don't come to close to me. Ha, ha."

Betty was stunned. Before she could say anything, Mrs. Cooney had already moved toward another group.

Betty asked her friends, "Is she the Gabrielle whom we thought was the dumbest student in our class?"

"Yes, she is that Gabrielle. Betty, you better watch your language. Many people think that she is the brightest girl in our class."

"What did she do?"

"She found a boyfriend while she was a student nurse and they married after her graduation. The boyfriend turned out to be a super nerd and a genius of programming. He started a software company and made billions. According to the rumor, his wealth is comparable to Bill Gates of Microsoft or Larry Ellison of Oracle."

One of her former friends said. "Betty, have you ever thought about the irony of this world? The dumbest student became a billionaire, and the brightest student stayed a poop nurse."

The person probably made the comment as a joke, but it truly stabbed her inner feelings. Betty left the meeting soon, and she decided that this town was not the place for her.

She was so upset about hearing her old derogatory nickname Poop-nurse that she did not notice the significance of the name Cooney at first. She felt the name seemed familiar but could not connect it to anything concrete. Then, she suddenly remembered who John Cooney was. He was a student who shared the same dormitory with her boyfriend, who later became her husband. John asked her for a date, but she refused his request because she felt he was creepy and weird. He had been tenaciously chasing and stalking her. Eventually, she had to ask her boyfriend to protect her from Cooney's pursuit. Because of the incident, her husband and Cooney severed their relationship completely. Even after finding out during a school reunion that Cooney became a billionaire, she did not regret her past action of abandoning the creepy Cooney and marrying her husband. However, she felt the insult and irony of Gabriel's marriage to Cooney.

Shortly after the reunion, she signed a contract with a traveling nurse company. The job of a traveling nurse was to serve as a staff nurse for a limited period, usually one to twelve months, in a hospital that had a temporary shortage of staff nurses. For instance, Florida was a place where all hospitals had seasonal fluctuations of demand for staff nurses.

Her job took her all over the country: one month in Sacramento, California, five weeks in Sedona, Arizona, three months in Denver, Colorado, and so on. She originally wondered how her husband would take her traveling around and her absence for irregular and long periods of time. It turned out that he had enjoyed the change of lifestyle and visited her often at her temporary homes in different cities. Both enjoyed these weekend mini-vacations. Betty took the situation for granted and renewed her contracts job after job. She took a six-month assignment in Okeechobee, Florida. Her husband visited her almost every weekend for the first month, but the frequency of his visits reduced gradually and after three months, he stopped his visits completely. He made various excuses. He said he was too busy to take a weekend off; he did not feel well; travel was too costly, etc.

Two weeks before the end of her six-month assignment, he dropped a bombshell on her. She received a certified letter from him. It said that he had already moved into his new girl friend's house. He wanted a divorce from her. If she did not agree to the divorce, she would receive their house and other favorable financial arrangements (in his opinion). If she would agree with the condition, she should sign the enclosed legal papers and return them to the address indicated. It was an attorney's address. His new address was nowhere in the letter.

They had been married for thirty-five years. She was devastated by both the divorce itself and the way her husband had informed her. She thought they had a much closer relationship. Apparently she was wrong. No, she could not accept that assumption. She would like to believe loneliness and the attraction of a new girlfriend overrode their relationship. Whatever the real cause, she had to accept the new situation. She thought about contesting the divorce, but it had drained her emotionally so much that she did not have the courage to deal with the uncertainty. After one week of crying and agony, she finally signed the legal papers and sent them back.

When she returned to her home, the house was well maintained, and almost nothing was missing. It seemed her former husband took only a few items with him when he moved out. Very soon, her neighbors visited her for consolation and gossiping. According to them, the girlfriend of her former husband was the young widow of a wealthy businessman and lived in a large mansion in Watertown, several miles away from her house. She could not bear to live in the house alone.

It was painful for her. Every item in the house reminded her of her former husband.

Within a month, she sold her house and decided to move to Florida. Fortunately, the hospital where she had worked before offered her a permanent position. After five years, she decided to retire. She bought and moved into a house in a nearby retirement community, where this author lived. Ever since, Betty has been living there peacefully and enjoying her life.

The author's original plan was to conclude this article at the time of Betty's retirement. When he finished his article, he showed it to Betty. She was perfectly happy about the contents. However, the author felt otherwise. He thought that he owed something more to the readers of the article. He felt obliged to present answers to several questions raised in the article. These questions are, for instance, where we stand now on the subject of the fecal transplant as a medical procedure. Do Chinese really use the yellow dragon soup even today? The author decided to add one more chapter to this story in order to address these questions.

Chapter 5: PM Colitis

Some folks believe that the medical profession has a tendency to talk about subjects normally avoided by others during their dinner meetings such as bed pans or urine samples. Even medical people try to avoid serious discussion about stools. The author could not find any serious study about fecal transplant colloquially referred to as *poop transplant*, during or before the first half of the twentieth century in medical journals in Western countries.

Around the late 1950s, there was a minor epidemic of pseudo-membranous entero-colitis (PM colitis), a type of inflammation of the large intestine, in the surgical wards in many hospitals. It usually occurred in post-operative patients who went through some kinds of colon or stomach surgery. Its symptoms were high fever and severe diarrhea. The seriousness of the disease was its alarmingly high fatality rate (74%) with no known effective treatment.

Surgeons from the University of Colorado and the Veteran's Administration Hospital together decided to do something about this epidemic. Since the disease happened in several types of operations, they thought the common factor among these patients was the antibiotic treatments they had received. These patients usually receive high dosages of a combination of multiple antibiotics in order to prevent infection. Therefore, doctors speculated that these antibiotics had killed the entire normal bacteria in the patient's gut that were helping a regular digestive process, and encouraged pathogenic bacteria to proliferate instead.

The doctors decided to reestablish the regular intestinal bacterial flora by injecting normal feces into the colons of the affected patients. They used a saline solution of feces from donors who had not received any antibiotic during the previous several months. Once they performed what they called a retention fecal enema, the patient recovered quickly. They repeated the same procedure successfully on three more patients. It was the first academically recognized research on fecal transplant, and its result was published in 1958. (Ref. 1)

It was a great discovery for patients who were suffering PM colitis. However, the doctors were not satisfied. They had simply demonstrated the efficacy of an unorthodox treatment. They wanted to know the detailed working mechanism of fecal enema over the unknown pathogen. They had concentrated their effort to identify the pathogen, namely the bacteria that caused the PM colitis. Once they identified the bacteria, a more orthodox treatment method could be devised easily, without relying on the psychologically repelling fecal enema.

The doctors monitored patients' fecal bacteria and discovered that bacteria called Micrococcus pyogenes (which were commonly referred to as Staphylococcus or Staph.) were abundant before the enema and completely disappeared after the enema. The doctors assumed that Staphylococcus was the pathogen of the PM colitis epidemic. They had tried hard to prove the hypothesis with various animal experiments, but could not prove it. (Ref.2)

Chagrined by PM colitis patients, medical researchers did not pay too much attention to the effectiveness of the fecal enema, but for the next twenty years they focused their effort on identifying the pathogen of PM colitis. Despite its known effectiveness, the fecal enema was not widely accepted for the treatment of PM colitis. Hundreds of patients suffered, and some died during this period without the benefit of the fecal enema. Nevertheless, PM colitis was considered to be an anomaly in the surgical wards.

Researchers focused their efforts on the identification of the pathogen for PM colitis. They proposed several candidates for the pathogen for PM colitis during the twenty year period between 1958 and

1978. The most popular one was the Staphylococcus, then Escherichia coli (E. coli) and Salmonella, etc. However, none was confirmed as the pathogen of PM colitis. During the same period, a few researchers had shown the effectiveness of the fecal transplant for the treatment of PM colitis, but the method never became widely accepted.

Due to the results of the high level of research, the search for the PM colitis pathogen was finally revealed in 1978. (Ref. 3) It was bacteria called Clostridium difficile (or C-diff), which had been discovered and given a different name as early as 1935. It turned out that the C-diff was fairly common and about two to five percent of the adult population carried C-diff in their colons. (Ref.4) C-diff infection would also take many different forms. Some persons who were C-diff infected had almost no symptoms. The other patients would have recurrent mild to moderate diarrhea, which resembled irritable bowel syndrome (IBS). These patients might consider that these symptoms were a normal part of their bowel behaviors.

Some other patients would have symptoms that could not be distinguished from colitis and were often diagnosed as idiopathic colitis (colitis with unknown cause). The severest infection could develop into PM colitis, or correctly, C-diff infection, when the natural protection of intestinal bacterial flora had been destroyed by the use of antibiotics. (Ref. 5) In this case, C-diff infection could be fatal, especially for already weakened post-operative patients. The standard treatment method for these severe cases of C-diff infection was the discontinuation of general purpose antibiotics and switching to carefully selected special purpose antibiotics such as vancomycin. (Ref. 6)

In 1983, again the fecal transplant was rediscovered as an effective alternative treatment method for PM colitis, which is now being referred to as C-diff infection. (Ref. 7) However, the fecal transplant was not adopted by the main line of medical professions. Many C-diff infected patients who were treated by the standard method had suffered a recurrence of the same disease after discharge from the initial treatment. This unsatisfactory condition continued for a long time, even today.

When the use of antibiotics became more common, it accelerated the emergence of more antibiotic-resistant bacteria. Many hospitals started having the experience of a large number of post-operative patients with C-diff infection or similar diseases because of the heavy usage of antibiotics. Around the year 2000, a new strain of C-diff which had strong resistance to antibiotics had emerged. The number of patients with severe C-diff infection started rising throughout the world, and the C-diff infection became a serious public health issue. By 2005, in the United States alone, approximately 3 million cases of diarrhea and colitis were caused by C-diff infection annually. The mortality rate (death ratio among the general population, rather than that among patients) is 1 to 2.5 %. (Ref. 8) In other words, 30,000 to 75,000 patients had died in 2005 alone in the United States due to C-diff infections.

Statistics are just numbers and have no emotion. But the lives of many former PM colitis patients were miserable. For instance, Mrs. Smith from Florida, who was a healthy and active eighty-seven-year-old woman, caught a cold and went to the hospital. It turned out to be pneumonia. One week later she was discharged from the hospital. She continued to take two different antibiotics at home. She became weak and short of breath, so two weeks later she had to go back to the hospital. Her pneumonia worsened. Doctors administered the same antibiotics. By the next day, she developed fever and diarrhea. She now had C-diff infection. Doctors discontinued two antibiotics and gave her three different antibiotics. After four weeks of various treatments her condition improved, so she was transferred to a nursing home. Her life in a nursing home was distressed and unbearable, because she had to wear diapers always and to use a wheelchair to get around. It was a typical problem of severe C-diff infection caused by antibiotic-resistant C-diff. The standard treatment for severe C-diff infection did not cure the disease, but it stabilized the disease into the manageable level of diarrhea. Furthermore, many patients experienced the recurrence of the full-fledged severe C-diff infection.

Because of heavy usage of antibiotics, antibiotic resistant C-diff infested almost all hospitals in U.S. So; all hospital patients became subjected to the exposure to these dreadful C-diff bacteria. They are spore-forming bacteria. When encountered in unfavorable environments, they enclose themselves into spores, which are hard shell capsules. They are heat-resistant and acid-resistant, which means they are immune to stomach acid. They survive against commonly used cleansers and disinfectants. They endur up to forty days on a hard surface even if the surface is wiped periodically by a cleanser. Regular hand-sanitizer is useless against them.

Therefore, many patients will catch C-diff in hospitals. In a hospital setting, bed rails, floors, windowsills, and toilets were cultured for C-diff bacteria, as well as the hands of hospital workers. According to one study, thirteen percent of patients who stayed up to two weeks acquired C-diff as did fifty percent of patients who stayed longer than four weeks. (Ref. 9)

Despite existence of many alarming signs for the infection of C-diff bacteria in hospitals, the medical establishment in the United States was slow to react. Especially in the treatment method of severe C-diff infection, the known effective treatment of fecal transplant was almost completely ignored.

References for Chapter Five

* Ref. 1: Eiseman B, Silen W, Bascom GS, and Kauvar AJ, "Fecal enema as an adjunct in the treatment of pseudomembranous enterocolitis", *Surgery*. 1958 Nov; 44 (5): 854-9. (No free public access. See Ref. 2)

* Ref. 2: http://www.twileshare.com/ uploads/784231.pdf) (Reprint of Ref. 1)

*Ref. 3: "Clostridium difficile and the aetiology of pseudomembranous colitis", by Larson HE, Price AB, Honour P, and Borriello SP (May 1978). *Lancet,* 311 (8073): 1063-6.

* Ref. 4: Ryan KJ, Ray CG (editor) (2004). *Sherris Medical Microbiology* (4th ed.) McGraw-Hill. Pp 322-4. ISBN0-8385-8529-9

* Ref. 5: "Infection with Clostridium difficile" by Centre for Digestive Diseases. http://www.cdd.au/pages/disease_info/clostridium_diffi cile.html.

* Ref. 6: "Colitis caused by Clostridium difficile: A review" by Weymann LH. A*m. J. Med. Technol.* 1982 Nov; 48(11), 927-34.

* Ref.7: "Relapsing clostridium difficile enterocolitis cured by rectal infusion of homologous feces" by Schwan A, Sjolin S, Trottestam U, and Aronson B. *Lancet*, 1983 Oct. 8; 2(8354) 845. (No free public access.)

* Ref. 8:"Clostridium difficile-- Associated Diarrhea" by Michael S. Schroder, Am Fam Physician, 2005 Mar;71(5): 921-928.

* Ref. 9: "Acquisition of Clostridium difficile by hospitalized patients: evidence for colonized new admissions as a source of infection." By Clabots CR, Johnson MM, Peterson LR, and Gerding DN. *J Infect. Dis.* 1992; 16:561-7.

Chapter 6:

Bureaucratic Obstacles

In Australia Dr. Thomas Borody, a gastroenterologist, and director of the Centre for Digestive Diseases, had established the Probiotic Therapy Research Centre in the year 2000. Its purpose was to provide an alternative treatment of fecal microbiota transplantation. In Scotland, Dr. MacConnachie from Gartnaval General Hospital started to provide fecal transplants in 2003 and successfully cured many C-diff infected patients by the end of 2011.

The adaptation of the fecal transplant or similar techniques in the United States lagged behind other developed countries. U.S. doctors were often discouraged from performing a fecal transplant by their partners or affiliated hospitals because of liability concerns and also bureaucratic hurdles of the impossibility of a billing procedure. In the United States, a snag in governmental protocol prevented even the research of the procedure.

For the fecal transplant to become widely accepted, it must be rigorously studied in a randomized clinical trial. If the trial were successful, the procedure would be recommended by professional societies and the Food and Drug Administration (FDA) would approve the procedure. Then health insurance companies would assign associated billing codes for the procedure, with which doctors would be able to request a reimbursement for fees.

Several doctors tried to apply for a grant for randomized clinical trials of the fecal transplant to the National Institute of Health (NIH). But they found out that NIH could approve a clinical trial only when the studied substance has to meet the qualification of an "investigational new drug (IND)" status by the FDA. However, the regulation states that the substance must be new drugs, devices, and new biological products such as vaccines and tissues. Unfortunately, the substance in this case was feces, which cannot receive the qualification as new biological products and do not belong in any categories. As a result, it could not get an IND status. There was no easy way around this simple bureaucratic hurdle. If the fecal transplants were a potentially big money maker, an army of lobbyists would be mobilized to change the regulation, but the fecal transplant had no pharmaceutical company to promote the procedure. So, U.S. researchers were handicapped compared to other countries to perform the fecal transplant, in addition to the fear of potential liability lawsuits.

There were thousands of former C-diff infected patients who were still suffering severe diarrhea, but they were not aware of the effectiveness of the fecal transplant. However, this condition gradually changed. In July 2010, the New York Times carried an article about a successful fecal transplant to cure the vicious C-diff infection, which Dr. Khoruts from the University of Minnesota performed. (Ref. 10) The article intended to describe a biome research, which was a new field of study of the entire species of microbes in the human body, and did not specifically emphasize the fecal transplant. But some patients noticed the article and demanded their doctors perform similar procedures. These demands apparently stimulated the status review of fecal transplant research. Several professional medical journals published reviews and guidelines in 2011 not only in the printed media, but also in a few blog sites that appeared on the Internet. Some were aimed toward physicians, and others were intended for laypersons, including a do-it-yourself guide for the fecal enema. Also, popular news media started showing interest in the subject. For instance, ABC broadcasted a TV program in July 2011; the Wall Street Journal had an article in October 2011, and the BBC televised a program on the fecal transplant in December 2011.

Among these popular news media presentations, the most influential one, in this author's opinion, was an article in December 2011 Scientific American. (Ref. 11) The article reviewed not only the status of the fecal transplant research in the U.S., but also pointed out the reason U.S. research was hindered, namely because of a bureaucratic protocol. It mildly blamed the U.S. government for blocking the research of this potentially most effective treatment method for C-diff infection.

Probably in response to the Scientific American article, the Center for Disease Control and Prevention (CDC) posted an article on its Web site on January17, 2012. It said:

It increasingly appears that fecal transplants are effective in treating recurrent C-diff infection. Though we await randomized controlled trials to confirm signs of efficacy, we at CDC are heartened by this potential treatment ⋯. We need to know more about fecal transplants and the role of a healthy microbiome to bring this to the bedside. To speed this process, CDC is working with other government agencies, the NIH, and FDA, to translate microbiome science into practical infection prevention ⋯. (Ref. 12)

The government finally admitted its shortcoming and started to do something, but very slowly. This author could not see any concrete action by the government until 2013. Meanwhile, more and more persons were infected by C-diff in hospitals. Many of them became desperate and begged their doctors to do something or anything to relieve their pain and suffering. Some brave doctors or patients started to perform the fecal transplant of their own accord.

For instance, Mrs. Catharine Duff had eight episodes of recurring C-diff infection beginning in 2005. Eventually, the recurrent C-diff infection became resistant to any known standard treatments. She had been suffering from constant pain and severe diarrhea. She had spent most of her time lying in bed without the energy to do anything. She eventually reached a point that she did not care anymore to live in such a condition. Then she found out about the fecal transplant. She asked doctors to perform the treatment. Some doctors had never heard of the fecal transplant. Other doctors knew of the procedure but refused to perform the treatment by themselves, because they could not get permission from their partners or affiliated hospitals.

As a desperate last measure, in March 2012 Mrs. Duff performed the fecal transplant using an enema in her house with the help of her husband as a donor and an injector. Within days, her pain stopped and no more diarrhea. Within a week, she recovered completely. She was so impressed by the effectiveness of the fecal transplant that she decided to help fellow sufferers who were affected with the same disease. She established

The Fecal Transplant Foundation in order to promote the fecal transplant. (Ref. 13) The foundation certified the doctors who would provide the fecal transplant for the treatment of C-diff infection.

While the number of recurrent C-diff infected patients in the U.S. was increasing, there was no significant improvement in the standard treatment. At the same time, the Internet and popular news media had been promoting and spreading the effectiveness of the fecal transplant against C-diff infection. For example, CNN broadcasted a TV program on fecal transplant in September 2012. The popularity and publicity did not change the majority of doctors and regulations by government agencies. Their major excuse was that there was no randomized clinical trial ever performed,. However, they did not admit that the existing U.S. policy practically banned the performance of such a study because there was no way to get funding from NIH.

This situation finally changed. In January 2013, The New England Journal of Medicine, one of the most respected medical journals in the world, published a paper. The paper described the result of a randomized clinical trial of the fecal transplant, performed in the Netherlands. (Ref. 14) Since the journal publisher had provided a pre-publication news release for mass media, these mass media published their articles at the same time as the official release date of the journal. For instance, the New York Times, Los Angeles Times,

The Boston Globe, CBS New, and Huffington Post, and other notable mass media simultaneously reported this curiously interesting subject: the fecal transplant.

Some news media had tried to distinguish themselves from others, so, they included their selected stories, in addition to the summary of the journal article. These headlines summarized their efforts along with the content of the research paper. The following are some actual headlines.

* Fecal transplants beat antibiotics for curing diarrhea caused by C-diff

* Self-Prescribed Fecal Transplant Saves Canadian Man's Life

* Fecal Transplant: They Work, the Regulations Don't

* Fecal Transplants Gaining Popularity! Still Gross!

* Fecal transplants show promise in infection fights

* Fecal transplants successful in treating intestinal ailment

*When Pills Fail, This, er, Option Provides a Cure

As a result of the onset of these attacks from mass media about obstacles and inaction with the government, the FDA/NIH finally started to take action. In early May 2013, they held a two-day workshop on "Fecal Microbiota for Transplantation". Because of the workshop, the Fecal Microbiota Transplantation (FMT) became the official name of the fecal transplant or colloquially referred to as poop transplant. The purpose of the workshop was "to bring together bench scientists, clinical researchers and those with regulatory expertise as well as other stakeholders to discuss various aspects of this quickly evolving field." (Ref. 15)

After the workshop, the government moved fairly quickly and issued changes to the regulations in the middle of 2013. Now, U.S. doctors can perform an FMT to treat recurrent C-diff infected patients without receiving permission from the FDA. Also, researchers can apply for grants for research on FMT to NIH. Some researchers have already engaged in several randomized clinical trials now.

It took more than a half-century from Betty's sad experience, but the fecal transplant is on the way to being a widely accepted treatment for C-diff infected patients. At present non-recurrent C-diff infected patients are not permitted to have FMT treatment.

References for Chapter Six

* Ref. 10: "How Microbes Defend and Define Us" by Carl Zimmer, *The New York Times*, July 12, 2010.

* Ref. 11: "Swapping Germs: Should Fecal Transplants Become Routine for Debilitating Diarrhea?" by Maryn McKenna, Scientific American, Dec. 2011.

* Ref. 12: http://blogs.cdc.gov/safehealthca re/2012/01/17/using-fecal-transplants-ttreat-recurrent-clostridium-difficile-infections-cdi/

* Ref. 13: http://thefecaltransplantfounda tion.org/founder-message/

* Ref. 14: "Duodenal infusion of donor feces for recurrent Clostridium difficile." By van Nood ,Vrieze A, Nieuwdorp M, uenties S, Zoetenddal EG, de Vos WM, Visser CE, Kuijper EJ, Bartelsman JF, Tijssen JG, Speelman P, Djkgraaf MG, and Keller JJ. N. Engl J Med 2013 Jan 31; 368(5): 407-15.

* Ref. 15: From an opening remark by Dr. Karen Midthun, at a workshop on FMT on May 2, 2013 at Bethesda, Maryland.

Chapter 7:

Chinese Medicine

In the frenzy of the news media about fecal transplant in early 2013, an article from the New York Times distinguished itself. In this author's opinion, the article had the most confusing headline, "When Pills Fail, This, er, Option Provides a Cure." (Ref. 16) It had the largest impact on popular media, especially on the Internet. The reason was that the article introduced a new terminology, **"Yellow Soup**," by quoting an obscure letter to the editor of a medical journal by Chinese doctors. (Ref. 17) They wrote that according to an ancient book, in traditional Chinese medicine, doctors had given patients soup made of feces by mouth to cure diarrhea in the fourth century. The soup was called **yellow soup**. In the U.S. people often show a high interest in any ancient remedy. The contrast between the latest development in medical science and the old Chinese traditional medicine stirred popular fascination. Since then most every article, including academic research papers, on the fecal transplant started to refer the old Chinese **yellow soup** as precedence for the fecal transplant.

Some astute readers may remember that Betty's Chinese friend told her that it was **yellow dragon soup**, based on information provided by a friend's grandfather, a practicing traditional Chinese doctor. This author also was intrigued by the difference and started research in to the classical Chinese medical books.

There were hundreds or thousands of books on classical Chinese traditional medicines, but, fortunately, only a few are widely used today. According to traditional Chinese doctors and pharmacists, human feces had been used in many applications. They wondered why Americans were making a big fuss about the use of feces of a human or other animals as medicine. The Chinese had been using almost everything on this earth as medicines: living or dead; animals, vegetables or minerals. The author was surprised to find a variety of the ingredients in traditional Chinese prescription. He found everything: chicken shit, rat pee, monkey brains, cow's stomach stones, mercury, sulfur, and so on. So feces and urine were not an exception.

An anonymous expert on traditional Chinese medicine in Japan claimed, "There are dozens of prescriptions using human excrement under several different names, but there was no **yellow soup** among them." Upon hearing that, this author decided to inspect the original Chinese texts, not their translations. He found the first reference to a Chinese medicine made of human feces in the book, titled *Handbook of Prescriptions for Emergencies* (*Zhouhou Jiuzufang*). Ge Hong (283 - 343 C.E.), who was a Taoist philosopher and the most famous alchemist in China wrote the book. (Ref. 18) He was a prolific writer and produced many volumes. The handbook includes thousands of various prescriptions for one hundred different diseases. Among them, there was only one prescription made of human excrement. It was called **yellow dragon soup**, not yellow soup, which was one of the many different methods to cure high fever. (Ref. 19) He also had believed that he could achieve physical immortality through alchemy, and he wrote a book that described a method to achieve immortality. He was a respected philosopher, and many Chinese and foreign scholars study his writings even today. However, his writings on medicine were not valued as much as those on philosophy, probably because of his belief in immortality.

This author also found a second classic book, containing the prescription of **yellow dragon soup.** It was *Essential Formulas for Emergencies [Worth] a*

Thousand Pieces of Gold (Beiji Qian Jin Yao Fang), written by Sun Simiao. (Ref. 20) He is a famous Chinese medicine doctor of the Sui and Tang dynasties. He was believed to have lived from 582 to 682 C.E. and was often called the King of Medicine because of his contribution. He also wrote *Supplement to the Formulas of a Thousand Gold Worth (Qian Jin Yi Fang)*. With these two books, he described a total of 7,300 recipes of medicines. Among these recipes, one mentioned **yellow dragon soup**.

He also defined what we call the Chinese Hippocratic Oath, which was still required reading by Chinese Physicians. The following is an excerpt from the text (Ref. 21)

A great physician should not pay attention to status, wealth, or age; neither should he question whether the particular person is attractive or unattractive, whether he is an enemy or a friend, whether he is a Chinese or a foreigner, or finally, whether he is uneducated or educated. He should meet everyone on equal grounds. He should always act as if he were thinking of his close relatives.

Chinese civilization is old and has a tradition of deep respect for their ancestors and their acts, which become precedents. Many kings and emperors attempted to preserve ancient knowledge by ordering the notable scholars to compile all known knowledge at that time in their special fields. One result of the attempts to preserve medical knowledge was a book, known as *Compendium of Materia Medica* (Ref. 22). The literal translation of the actual title is *Principles and Species of Roots and Herbes (Bencao Gangmu),* and Li Shizhen (1518 - 1593) wrote the massive book.

He was one of the greatest Chinese physicians, polymaths, scientists, herbalists, and acupuncturists in history. He was also considered to be a great scientific naturalist since he devised a proper method of classification of herb components. (Ref. 23) His compendium consisted of fifty plus volumes and contained almost 2,000 distinct herbs, including almost 400 which had been newly discovered by him. It described eleven thousand different prescriptions for more than eight thousand diseases. Among them, he quoted four different recipes of human stool-based medicines from different classic texts. All four were used for the cure of high fever diseases, but their production methods were different.

Interestingly, Li Shizhen did not mention Ge Hung and his handbook nor Sun Simiao's *Essential Formulas*, even though Li read more than 800 other medical reference books. Li described **yellow dragon soup** in detail and also listed its variations. According to him, people called the yellow dragon soup by different names such as spirit of stool, recycled water, and yellow human excrement. However, he did not include the name **yellow soup** as quoted by the New York Times.

Based on the above result, this author must conclude that **yellow soup** was a mistranslation or a misquotation of **yellow dragon soup**, which the grandfather of Betty's friend mentioned.

Since the Chinese had known that human stool could be used for a medication to cure the disease, does it mean that they had been using the medicine? If so, how widely was it used? It is not easy to obtain accurate data, if it exists, but this author encountered an interesting example on the internet.

A Japanese person asked for a traditional Chinese medicine adviser.

"When I had severe diarrhea, a trusted friend of mine, who was Chinese, but not a doctor, gave me a powdered medicine It did not work, and made my diarrhea worse. After I had checked the dictionary, I found that its Japanese name, "Jin-chu-ou" was equivalent to "Ren-zhong-huang" in Chinese, and it meant medicine made of human stool. Can I sue him for misrepresentation?"

An adviser replied, "You probably cannot, because you had trusted a non-medical person and asked for medical advice. The person did his best, but it turned out to be wrong. It was his honest mistake, but the fault was your side: You tried to extract medical advice from an amateur, instead of from a doctor of traditional Chinese medicine."

This anecdote indicates that a traditional Chinese medicine which is made from human stool is easily available and still reasonably popular, even though the correct usage may require a professional judgment.

How about the real **yellow dragon soup**, is it still in use? The answer is a qualified yes. Remember Betty's friend's grandfather. He used the **yellow dragon soup** sixty years ago. Since traditional Chinese medicine rarely changes its methodology, it is very likely that the **yellow dragon soup** is still in use at least in China and Chinese communities in foreign countries, where traditional doctors are in practice.

How about other Far Eastern countries where traditional Chinese medicine is widely accepted, is there any **yellow dragon soup**? In Japan, there exists a traditional medicine called **yellow dragon soup**, but its ingredient does not contain any human excrement. In Korea, the answer is a definite yes. It is a traditional medicinal wine, called "Ttongsul (Dung Sake)." Heo Jun (1613) originally described the wine in the oldest traditional Korean medicine book, *Treasure Mirror of Eastern Medicine (Dongui bogam)*. The wine is not widely used nowadays, but it is still available from the underground market. (Ref. 24) Based on limited information, it seems to resemble one of the four known varieties of Chinese **yellow dragon soup**.

References for Chapter Seven

* Ref. 16: "When Pills Fails, This, er, Option Provides a Cure" by Denise Grady. *The New York Times*, January 16, 2013.

* Ref. 17: "Should We Standardize the 1700-Years-Old Fecal Microbiota Transplantation?" (Letter to the Editor) by Faming Zhang, Wensheng Luo, Yan Shi, Zhining Fan, and Guozhong Ji, Am J Gastroenterology 2012: 107:1755. (No abstract, no free public access.)

* Ref. 18: http://zh.wikipedia.org/zh/ %E8%91%9B%E6%B4%AA (Chinese language site on Ge Hong.)

* Ref. 19: http://wikisource.org/wiki/ %E8%82%98%E5%BE%8C%E5%82%99%E6%80%a 5%E...(Chinese text of *Handbook of Prescriptions for Emergencies*.)

* Ref. 20: http://zh.wikipedia.org/wiki/ %E5%AD%99%E6%80%9D%E9%82%88. (This is Chinese language site of Sun Simiao. From there, you can go to the original Chinese text of *Essential Formulas for Emergencies*...)

* Re. 21: http://en.wikipedia.org/wiki/ Sun_Simiao

* Ref. 22: http://en.wikipedia.org/wiki/ Compendium_of_Materia_Medica. (From here, go to Chinese translation site, and then you can access the original Chinese full text.)

* Ref. 23: http://en.wiki[edia.org/wiki/ Li_Shizhen

* Ref. 24: http://en.wikipedia.org/wiki/ Ttongsul

Chapter 8:

Yellow versus Brown

When I thought I finished this book, I brought my manuscript to Betty and gave it to her for reviewing. A few days later I visited her.

"Hi Betty, how's everything with you?"

"Thank you, I am OK, so far so good."

"What do you think about my fecal transplant book?"

"First, I was surprised at its length. I thought you would write an article of your normal length, just like your short story in our community newsletter. Looks like this is a book, and not an article."

"It started out as an article, but my muse drove me to keep going. Eventually, I have to stop the story. Otherwise, I would write about the whole history of

Chinese medicine, which has little relation to your story."

Betty said, "But you included one chapter on Chinese medicine, didn't you?"

"Yes, I did. I wanted to clarify that your story of yellow dragon soup was correct, and the New York Times' yellow soup was not. The name yellow soup is an error in translation or quotation."

"Thank you. That indicates at least that I did not cook up the story. But you made up a good story. I never thought that you would be able to compose a full-length book from my tiny anecdote."

"It is not a full-length book, but more likely a booklet. It is about 15,000 words long, and a full-length book has to have a minimum of 80,000 words. Returning to my original question, how do you feel about the contents of this book? Does it depict the general feeling of your experience?"

Betty seemed annoyed by my new question. "My general feeling? I think yes. This book describes my feeling accurately enough, but lots of details were different from what happened. Even though I don't mind these differences, I wanted to correct one thing. It would make a crucial point for the validity of my story."

"What is it?"

"I did not use distilled water but used a saline solution. Any nurse or doctor knows that we do not inject distilled water into a patient's body. So, they would not believe your story at all. Also, I did not use a ball injector for the enema."

"I am sorry, Betty. I apologize. I researched lots, but I hardly gained any knowledge about the details of the actual practice. If you did not use a ball injector, then did you use a plastic bag? Based on my research, that was the only alternative method. When I wrote the scene, I had to make an arbitrary choice of a ball injector."

Betty smiled and said, "No, the use of disposable plastic bags came much later. In my time, we had to reuse every bit of equipment with repeated sterilization by baking in an autoclave. I used equipment called Monel. I had no idea what the name meant or where it came from."

It was my turn to show off. I said, "Betty, I know that. As a former engineer, I am familiar with the name and know what that means. It is the name of a special metal, which has strong resistance to corrosion. It is a kind of super stainless steel. So the name of the equipment came from its material. What does your Monel look like?"

"I never knew that Monel was the name of the material. Thank you Yashi. Our Monels were like a beaker with a spout at the bottom. We had several different sizes of Monels. I used a quart size Monel. I cut about 6 feet of 1/4 inch diameter rubber tube from the master spool. Again, we did not have plastic tubing at that time. I pushed one end of the tube onto the spout of the Monel and a metal nozzle to the other end. Then I attached a metal clip to the middle of the tube to control the flow of fluid. I have forgotten details about the incident, and this is the best I can do now. I am hoping that these minor details will enhance the trustworthiness of my story."

"Thank you Betty for the correction. The Monel improves the validity of our story. Now I want to ask you about your thoughts on the general state of the fecal transplant in the United States."

"I feel good about the fact that the fecal transplant has finally become available to C-diff patients, even with some restriction. I hope that many more hospitals and doctors will adopt this effective treatment method for patients suffering severe diarrhea from C-diff infection. One thing I occasionally think about is my role in this treatment. If I were much stronger and had fought back against incessant teasing, and if I had promoted the use of fecal transplant from the beginning, lives of thousands of patients could have been saved. But I was young and inexperienced in survival in this competitive world. I was too busy saving my sanity and had no time to think about suffering patients."

"Wow! You still maintain the spirit of Nightingale. Don't blame yourself. You did your best. In every field, there are pioneers, whose actions were not rewarded. As you mentioned, this is a cutthroat world and often villains win, and good persons lose.

How do you feel about the action or non-action of our government on the problem of C-diff and the fecal transplant?"

Betty was silent a few seconds and said, "I am angry at our government, especially the lack of leadership. Thousands of people were dying every year, due to hospital acquired C-diff, but they did not take any positive actions. We had a known effective cure, but they ignored the fact. If the government took action in the year 2000, when the antibiotic-resistant strain of C-diff appeared, we would have saved the lives of more than a million people. Progress in our medical practice heavily depends on commercial companies, because of our market economy system. Commercial companies ignore any medical practices that do not produce a profit. So, the government has to take the initiative for the development of low-cost, effective treatment methods such as fecal transplant. However, our government agencies acted like any other commercial companies. They ignored a low cost, highly effective treatment method, while thousands of patients were dying every year. I am sorry, Yashi. I burst out my favored soap box opinion. Now I am too old to be involved in any politics, so I should not have said anything. I just want to live the rest of my life peacefully."

"I agree with you about the government's attitude, but we, poor peasants, can do very little to change that. We will put aside politics and come back to the subject of our book. Are there any questions or additional comments about our book?" I said.

"Yes, you had said that you would resolve the question of yellow and brown soup discrepancy, but so far you never mentioned it again in the book."

"Oh, that. It was so obvious to me that I forgot. In the Far Eastern countries, namely China, Korea, and Japan, human stool was always referred to as yellow or gold in color. I was surprised that the stool was brown in this country. To illustrate our ignorance, I will tell you one anecdote from my boyhood." The following is my story.

I was about twelve years old. The time was the 1940s when the U.S. and Japan were in the state of war. We knew we were fighting with Whiteman, but none of us had ever seen any Whiteman. So, everything about Whiteman was a mystery to us, and we had often questioned many aspects of their physical characteristics without getting any valid answers. On that particular day, we had a big argument in our classroom during recess. Several pupils had heated discussions. The subject of discussion was the color of stool.

One boy asked, "We are fighting with people of the white race, and we are the yellow race. When we shit, we see that our shit is yellow. So would these white guys make white shit?'

"No, they also will shit yellow like us," one boy said.

"No, you are wrong. Why we call them Whiteman, because they lack the pigment to block the sun's rays. Everything they produce will be of no color, namely their shit is white."

The wisest boy in our class said, "Both of you are wrong. Did you see the shit of lions?" Nobody answered, so he continued. "When I went to the Zoo, I saw a lion that was defecating. It produced black droppings. Lion eats meat and Whiteman eats meat, so their droppings must be black."

Since he was the smartest kid in our class and used the word defecating, he intimidated everyone and stopped the discussion.

The story amused Betty, "I did not know your stool color was yellow."

"I need to make a correction. When I arrived in the United States fifty plus years ago, I was surprised to learn that people referred to stool color as brown, not black, or yellow. Eventually, I started to produce brown stool myself. Then, I finally had an answer to the question of my boyhood. The color of the stool depends on the food we eat. In my old country, people eat rice as the main staple, and they produce stool of a yellow color. In this country, wheat and meat are the main staples. Thus, their stool becomes brown."

Betty was surprised and said, "Do you know what you are saying? You are implying that the stool transplant between different ethnic groups may not work. It could be potentially a big problem in the future of the fecal transplant."

"Well, I am not a medical doctor, but I think it can be."

"Now our book could make some contribution to the progress of medical science. So, I can show it proudly to other people. Thank you, Yashi."

"Thank you, Betty for sharing your experience with me and our readers."

Chapter 9:
Missed Opportunity

As mentioned previously, the official name of the fecal transplant became the fecal microbiota transplantation (FMT). On one hand, it showed progress on standardizing the name of the procedure, which is called the fecal transplant in this book. People had called the fecal transplant many different names: poop transplant, fecal enema, fecal transplant, fecal implant, fecal transfusion, fecal bacteriotherapy, fecal flora reconstitution, retention fecal enema, stool transplant, probiotic therapy, human probiotic infusion (HPI), human probiotic insufflation, restoration of human bowel flora, rectal infusion of homologous feces, duodenal infusion of donor feces, intestinal microbiota transplantation (IMT), etc.

On the other hand, this author dislikes the choice of the name *fecal microbiota transplantation* based on the following three grounds. Firstly, adopting a new name violates the tradition of honoring precedence. Secondly, the intentional avoidance of the name *fecal transplant* could be interpreted as the government wanting to disguise their missteps of the handling of the fecal transplant and to conceal the preventable death of thousands of C-diff patients. Thirdly, fecal microbiota transplantation could be a misnomer since we do not know yet whether a fecal transplant is transplanting fecal microbiota or transplanting a single species or a specific group of microorganisms. However, the reason this author has kept using the name *fecal transplant* throughout this book is not his disfavor of the name FMT. He thought that the intended readers of this book would feel the sound of the phrase *fecal transplant* familiar to them.

A remaining major question is, where will the fecal transplant go from here? This author believes that the next major step will be the treatment of a newly infected, not recurrent, C-diff patient with a fecal transplant. Why does the patient have to suffer unnecessary pain and the agony of a high fever and diarrhea while doctors are satisfying the current FDA requirement of proving the ineffectiveness of the present standard treatment procedure of the disease? The FDA should allow doctors to administer fecal transplant as soon as the C-diff infection is detected, without waiting for recurrence of the disease.

The second major step in the progress of the fecal transplant will be the introduction of a licensing system for the administration of fecal enemas by non-medical and semi-medical personnel, such as nurses, nursing aides, medical technicians, and enema specialists, without a doctor's involvement. This idea is controversial and will be opposed by the medical establishment. However, this author believes that such a bold movement is necessary to face a steadily increasing number of C-diff patients in nursing homes and long-term care units where many of the elderly in the aging U.S. population will eventually settle. Otherwise, we will repeat the same mistakes as in the initial stage of the fecal transplant procedures. Many C-diff patients in elder care facilities will suffer preventable pain, agony, and even death. We seemed to have successfully managed the hospital-acquired C-diff infection, but now the problem has moved to nursing homes and other facilities for elder care. These institutions are chronically understaffed and under-budgeted. They will not be able to handle the ever-increasing number of C-diff infected patients. We need a low cost, effective treatment to face this crisis. Fortunately, the fecal enema is easy to perform, and its associated cost is low. The only missing element is the personnel to perform the procedure in a timely fashion to many patients. The solution will be supplying a large number of enema specialists, whom we could train within a short time with minimum cost. The CDC and NIH should promote the idea in order to reestablish their reputation that was badly damaged by dealing with the fecal transplant development. In our economic system, commercial companies will not engage in unprofitable activities, even though those activities would be beneficial to all mankind. Unfortunately, the fecal transplant is one such procedure. Our only hope is to press the government for action.

At present, there are two attention-getting topics in the field of fecal transplants. One is a supply of standardized fecal specimens. In 2012, two graduate students of MIT, Mark Smith in microbiology and James Burgess in business management started a non-profit organization called OpenBiome. (Ref: 25) It was the first public stool bank, which supplies pre-screened and pre-processed stool specimens to hospitals and clinics for FMT treatment for C-diff patients. OpenBiome also acts as a research, analysis, and data collection organization for FMT, in order to expand our knowledge on FMT and underlying characteristics of the human biome. It is a commendable enterprise and will contribute to the advancement of FMT procedures as well as the expanded application of FMT far beyond the cure of C-diff patients. One of the potential stumbling blocks will be the validity of its operating hypothesis: the existence of the standardized stool, which could be used universally for all C-diff patients.

There are already some signs of invalidity of this hypothesis. Let think about a hypothetical case: a donor of the stool belongs to an ethnic group, and the patient belongs to another ethnic group. Furthermore, their dietary habits are completely different. In this case, is the stool of a donor compatible with a patient? For instance, is the stool of a vegetarian compatible to an Inuit patient who eats almost no vegetables? How about the age difference, can adult stool be usable on an infant patient? We can easily address the compatibility problem as long as researchers are open-minded and diligent. Until such a time, we have to be cautious about the universal application of the standard stool specimen to all C-diff patients.

The second popular topic is the oral administration of FMT in a form of pill or syrup. Since this form of FMT implementation has the potential for commercial product development, several companies have already started working on the process. The contents of oral medications could be unprocessed, semi-processed (frozen), or purified stool. From a patient's point of view, it is better to have the choice of an enema or oral medication. There was an anecdotal example of the administration of pills containing unprocessed stool to patients in the 1950s without notifying the patient of its contents. Under the present policy, the patient has to be notified, and the patient has to consent with the administration of the pill. So the effectiveness of an unprocessed stool pill would be doubtful, due to the patient's psychological rejection. Probably the most acceptable type of pills would contain a purified stool, which is cultivated in petri-dishes, not by direct extraction from a human. This author predicts that several different FMT pills will be available for clinical use within a few years, but he wishes that the fecal enema would become the main treatment method for the C-diff patients. He believes that it is the easiest, the least repulsive psychologically, and also the cheapest form of FMT implementation. In reality, the most accepted form of the implementation will be determined by the patients' preference, selection by insurance companies, and the effectiveness of advertisements for commercial products.

****

I thought that I completed this book at this point and was ready to publish it. When I received a proof copy from the printer for the final check of book contents, I showed it to Betty.

She said, "It is fine, I have nothing to correct or to change in content." However, she did not hand me a copy, and she held it tight. After a few seconds, she said, "It may not be your concern, but I have to tell someone. Recently an old friend of mine told me that my ex-husband died several months ago. I hated him because of what he did to me. When I heard the details on the circumstances of his death, I had a mixed feeling. I felt joy of revenge against his new wife, relief of the closure from the past, and regret for a missed opportunity. He apparently had colon cancer. Doctors operated on him successfully, and they removed all the cancer cells. During his recovery process, some complication occurred. He developed a high fever and severe diarrhea. Within a week, he was dead despite the best efforts of his doctors. The cause of his death was PM colitis. Do you believe those bumpkin doctors in that backward country? They were fifty years behind us. PM colitis! Did they ever hear of C-diff? He and his wife had been staying at her villa in the Caribbean country when he was struck by the cancer. So he was operated on by the best doctors in that country. If I was informed about his illness and associated complications, I would have flown to the country and would have performed fecal transplant. It was another missed opportunity for me! That was my life story: continuously, one missed opportunity after another missed opportunity." She paused a few seconds.

I did not know of any other missed opportunity in her life, but I kept my mouth shut and waited until she became calm.

After a few seconds, she became herself and said, "Can I keep this copy?"

I was surprised by the sudden change of the situation. It was a proof copy, which I intended to send back to my printer. I said, "I'd rather you not keep this copy. I will give you a complete book when I publish it."

"No, I want this unpublished copy because it is incomplete. Once you publish this book, anyone can purchase it. But this unpublished version is unique, and nobody will be able to acquire it. In the public's point of view, this version of the book does not exist. I think it would symbolize my experience with fecal transplant. The public does not recognize me, but nobody had the same experience I had, as the first performer of the fecal transplant. Please, can I keep this copy?"

I was unable to understand her logic, but I dared not say no. So, I left her house without the proof copy. I needed an excuse for the printer as to why I could not send back the corrected proof copy. Later that day I wrote to my printer that I decided to add one more chapter to the book. I had to postpone the publication of the book until I sent in the manuscript of the added chapter. I thought this would make Betty's copy unique since all the published copies would have an extra chapter.

Reference for Chapter Nine

Ref: 25: http://en.wikipedia.org/wiki/ OpenBiome

Chapter 10: FDA's Role

If the fecal transplant had been widely accepted in the early 1960s as a standard treatment for PM colitis, and C-diff infection at later dates, we could have prevented the emergence of the antibiotic resistant strain of C-diff bacteria. Even after the appearance of a new strain, we still had a chance. If the fecal enema had been the standard treatment for antibiotic-resistant C-diff infection, we would have prevented the deaths of almost one million C-diff patients,.

What hindered earlier adaptation of fecal transplants for the treatment of PM colitis and C-diff infection? The commonly accepted theory is the marketing economy. Since the fecal transplant had no profit potential for new investment, no pharmaceutical company was interested. We cannot blame commercial companies for that. It is natural under the marketing economy, namely the capitalistic economic system. No commercial company would invest in the development of a new medicine or new treatment method if there were no chance to recover the original investment and also make any profit.

However, an epidemic disease is a public health issue, not a commercial problem. If you like it or not, or whether your economy is a capitalistic or socialistic system, a new killer disease will appear and cause major disruptions in public health and also the economy. Regardless of the opportunity of making lots of profits or not, we have to prepare for such a disease. We need a treatment method and/or a vaccine for a potential major killer of many people. Currently, we treat a public health issue as an annoyance or a nuisance. When budget cuts come, public health is one of the first things to be reduced.

What will be the solution? The answer is a change to the present new drug and new treatment approval system. How should it be changed? There are several options to choose. For instance, this author's idea is to allow human patients as test agents for small-scale trial for new drugs and new treatments for which no profit potential exists. However, there will be no further discussion here on the subject since it is outside of the scope of this article.

While I was writing this article in the middle of October 2014, a panic due to the Ebola epidemic seized the United States. Ebola was discovered in 1976, in what is currently the Republic of Congo, but it had been considered to be a rare tropical disease, existing in a remote African region. In December 2013, an Ebola outbreak occurred in a small village in Guinea, a West African country. The disease spread quickly in West Africa. Ebola has a fatality rate of about 70%, but there is no effective treatment. In the United States, an official from the Centers for Disease Control and Prevention (CDC) assured us. In late July, they said that it was a very remote possibility that a traveler from West Africa could carry the Ebola virus to the U. S.

On August 8, 2014, when the death toll of Ebola reached the 1,000 mark, the World Health Organization (WHO) declared Ebola to be a global public-health emergency. About two months later, Mr. Thomas Eric Duncan, a Liberian, arrived in the U.S. with Ebola virus. He was treated at Dallas' Texas Health Presbyterian Hospital, which was supposed to be the top-level hospital in Texas. Not only did Mr. Duncan die, but two nurses who treated Mr. Duncan caught the disease and became Ebola patients. Unfortunately, these two nurses traveled before their infection was discovered. There was a possibility of spreading the disease to several hundred people. These two nurses had followed protocol set by the CDC, but they contracted the Ebola virus.

Our most trusted CDC did not know how to handle the Ebola epidemic. This distrust and ignorance about Ebola were the major causes of panic. Eventually, the panic subsided, but the experience demonstrated our unpreparedness against difficult-to-treat diseases.

We were lucky, because a terrorist organization such as Al-Qaeda or Muslim fanatics like ISIS had not discovered the tactics of using Ebola as a weapon for the fight against the United States. Imagine! A couple of dozens of suicide volunteers who were intentionally infected with Ebola arrive in the United States. Since their travel schedules could be carefully planned to coincide with Ebola's incubation period, they do not show any symptom of the disease. These disease carriers travel freely, and they scatter around the U.S. Within three weeks; they become ill and spread the disease all around the country. What a mess we would be in! It could be the repeat of the 1918 influenza pandemic, which killed 50 to 100 million people worldwide.

These incidents indicate that the public health problem could also be a national security issue, and the government has a responsibility to get ready for such an attack. Many people are willing to increase the defense budget, mainly weapon development, even during a tight budget period, but they are neglecting a public health issue. Development of vaccines and effective treatment methods for new killer diseases is a national security issue. So, the government has to prepare for them. As mentioned before, private companies will not engage in such nonprofit activities. We spend lots of money for the study of chronic diseases, but these are potentially money making opportunities or private companies. Let them be left to private companies, and have governmental agencies keep their emphasis on the public health diseases, namely the prevention of epidemics and pandemics.

On October 25, 2014 the New York Times carried an article titled, "Ebola Vaccine, Ready for Test, Sat on the Shelf: Lack of Market Stalled Drug's Development." (Ref. 26) According to the article, Dr. Thomas W. Geisbert, from the University of Texas Medical Branch in Galveston, created an Ebola vaccine about ten years ago. But it stayed at a prototype stage and never developed a marketable product because as he summarized, "There has never been a big market for Ebola vaccines."

This author's initial reaction was the same as before. Our economic system, which relies on a marketing force, prevented the further development of this obviously beneficial product for all mankind. How can we correct this situation? The most obvious answer is to change our economic system. But that seems to be unrealistic and impossible. This author had a conviction that there must be an easier and simpler solution. He investigated further and eventually found a solution.

The same article on the Ebola vaccine quoted the comment from Dr. James E. Crowe, Jr., the director of a vaccine research center at Vanderbilt University. He said that academic researchers who developed a prototype drug or vaccine that worked in animals often encountered a "biotech valley of death" in which no drug company will help them cross the finish line. According to him, the total cost to bring a vaccine to market will range between $1 billion and $1.5 billion. Nobody will invest such money unless the return is much higher than the investment. The bottleneck is the high cost differential between a research prototype and its marketable product. A major part of the cost is the clinical testing of the product in order to meet FDA requirements.

Why is the FDA approval procedure so costly? There is an interesting historical background for that. It all started with the Thalidomide Incident in the late 1950s. A German company, Grumenthal, marketed a miracle drug, called Contergan, which contained thalidomide, for morning sickness for pregnant women, and a cure for insomnia and headache. It was marketed worldwide, but, unfortunately, the drug had a severe side effect. It affected fetus development and produced babies with deformed and sometimes missing limbs. It was estimated about 10,000 babies with deformed limbs were born, and about 50% of them survived worldwide. The exception was the United States. The FDA refused to approve thalidomide for marketing and distribution, even though a U.S. agent of the drug applied for the permission six times. However, a large quantity of the drug was distributed in U.S. for testing purposes. As a result, a total of seventeen children with thalidomide-induced malformations were born. It was considered to be the success story of the FDA. The U.S. Congress also took action to prevent the recurrence of a similar tragedy. The result was The Kefauver-Harris Amendments of 1962, which was a supplement to the already existing Food, Drug and Cosmetic Act of 1938. It represented a revolution in FDA regulatory authority. The major new steps taken were as follows:

1. New drug development was rewarded with a product patent, rather than those for process. It allows a company to monopolize the new drug.

2. New drug manufacturers had to provide evidence of which proposed drugs were both safe and effective, and were proven by adequate and well-controlled clinical investigations conducted by qualified experts.

3. Manufacturers had to maintain records of adverse events associated with drugs and report these promptly to the FDA.

4. New drugs required an affirmative decision by the FDA before marketing. Approval would not be automatic anymore. Before the amendments, all applications were automatically approved within sixty days of their filing, unless the FDA objected to it.

5. New drugs were made available only through a prescription.

These changes were considered to make new drugs safer and more effective and also reduce health care cost. Unfortunately, the reality has generated many unexpected results during the past fifty years.

Reference for Chapter Ten:

* Ref. 26: "Ebola Vaccine, Ready for Test, Sat on the Shelf: Lack of Market Stalled Drug's Development." By Denise Grady, *The New York Times*, October 24, 2014.

Chapter 11:
New Drug Problems

One of the adverse effects of the new changes was a costly and lengthy approval process for new drugs and medical devices. For instance, a 2006 study indicated the cost to bring a new drug to market to be anywhere from five hundred million dollars to two billion dollars. (Ref. 27)

At the same time, the waiting time for new drug approval was increased from seven months, before the Kefauver-Harris amendments in 1962, to an average of 7.3 years by 1998. Following the AID/HIV epidemic, public pressure forced the FDA to amend its practices. They introduced an expedited approval of drugs for life-threatening diseases and expanded pre-approval access to drugs for patients with limited treatment options. However, most of the new drugs still had to exprience the normal approval process, which would cost nearly a billion dollars with a waiting period of an average of seven plus years.

Another unexpected result of the 1962 amendments was the price of drugs. Since the new FDA regulations allowed monopoly of the drug, the price of many drugs increased. The best-known example is the price of the drug called Makena, which had already been on the market for almost five decades. Its price increased from approximately ten dollars to fifteen hundred dollars in 2001 after the FDA regulated its marketing. However, it was reduced later, to some degree due to public pressure.

The present method of new drug approval is far from ideal. However, how to change it is a big question. When this author searched for an answer to the question on the Internet, surprisingly, he found many different suggestions. His conclusion, drawn from these different answers, is that many scholars and stakeholders were aware of the imperfectness of the present system, but there were many disagreements among them about how they should change it. At present, the FDA is a large, complex organization and consists of fifteen different divisions with nine thousand employees. They monitor and process one trillion dollars worth of products each year. (Ref. 28) For this reason, any attempt to reorganize the agency would be a formidable task.

There have been many attempts to improve and change the FDA since the 1962 Kefauver-Harris amendments. Congress introduced three separate amendments and nine different acts into the FDA. The last Congressional attempt to change the agency was the FDA Modernization Act of 1997. It was not a major change, but simple codification of various procedures already practiced. It may be a good time to attempt a true modernization of the FDA after the fiasco of the Ebola epidemic. Unfortunately, such a prospect is not likely under the current political situation. The only reasonable expectation is a minor tweaking of the existing procedures.

The problem we have now is caused by how we approach the new drug approval process. The underlying philosophy of the current procedure is that one method fits all cases. A new drug for a disease , which affects hundreds of patients, and another drug for a chronic disease, which afflicts millions of patients have to go through the same costly and lengthy approval procedures. We need a quicker and simpler procedure for a drug which will be used for a small number of patients. Such a procedure could be a streamlined version of the expedited approval procedure used for HIV drugs. In essence, the new drug approval procedure should be matched with the time, money, number of patients and nature of the disease. An approval process for a drug for a smaller market should be different from that of a drug that has the potential of large profits.

Another needed change in the basic philosophy of the approval process is the relaxation of safety requirements for selected cases. As we learned a lesson from the case of Ebola: we have to prepare a defense against a potential epidemic of a certain kind of rare disease. Some rare diseases have a small number of patients, only a few hundred worldwide, but the fatality rate is very high, and the disease is highly contagious, such as Ebola. As the front line of defense against these diseases, we have to bring research results of treatment methods and vaccines to the field as quickly as possible to prevent a wider spread of the disease. If no other alternative method exists in these cases, a high risk and less effective treatment/vaccine are acceptable. We already practiced this procedure for Ebola. An experimental drug ZMapp was used to treat eleven Ebola patients. We should adopt this type of approach as part of the formal approval procedure for certain types of drugs and diseases.

The results of Zmapp were uncertain. Some patients recovered and some didn't. An official conclusion was: "Its effectiveness was statistically not significant (to draw any conclusion)." This statement implies that the researcher who made it applied conventional criteria to judge the efficacy of Zmapp results. He should have used a different criterion for small sample experiments. There are many analytical methods to judge small sample experiments in other fields of science and technology, such as weapon testing, space exploration, weather forecasting, fluid dynamics, cosmology, etc.

To reduce costs and shorten the waiting period for the new drug approval process, we need a major revolution in our way of thinking about the process. It is impossible to perform the currently implemented procedure for drugs against a disease affecting a small number of patients, because there would not be enough patients, time, or money to perform the full-fledged approval procedure, which includes safety tests, randomized clinical tests, double-blind tests, etc. We need an alternative method. We have to substitute these lengthy and costly clinical tests with nonclinical means. We should search for substitutes in other fields of science –where real experiments were impossible to perform. They heavily rely on theoretical analysis, computer simulation, mathematical modeling, etc., and they achieve considerable success without real experiments and with a small number of test samples. We should explore this method and use a small number of human patients for test subjects. To achieve this goal, we need a better understanding of placebo effects and small sample experiment theories. If we had sufficient understanding of these two fields, we could eliminate or reduce the randomized, double-blind clinical tests and other expensive, lengthy clinical tests. This kind of study seems outside the scope of NIH, but this is vitally important for the future of medicine. Otherwise, the cost of medical care will bankrupt us.

Another area of study, which will have a drastic impact on any new drug approval procedure, is the requirement of the efficacy confirmation and failure analysis of clinical test results. When a new experimental drug is administered to a patient, a researcher should treat the opportunity as a precious moment because the researcher may not have any other chance to repeat a similar experiment. All possible data that have any connection to the drug should be collected and analyzed. By this analysis, we could prove or disprove the working hypothesis of the drug, namely the efficacy confirmation and failure analysis. The number of patients who will be exposed to the new drug should be minimized by the intensive analysis of available clinical data.

Both methodologies are commonly practiced in the engineering filed, but rarely applied in medicine. When a new drug is proposed, researchers have some idea as to why the drug is effective and how it works. When the drug is administered to a patient, the result is positive, negative, or uncertain. In any case, the researcher should pursue the cause: success, failure, or uncertainty of results. This will deepen the understanding of the working mechanism of the drug and may help discover selection criteria for the type of patients on which the drug can be effective. In the case of a blood transfusion, the selection of a patient and blood matching is routine, but it is rarely practiced with other medications or treatments. The matching process would reduce, or even eliminate, any unexpected side effects. In essence, we need a completely new approach in order to reduce the cost and shorten the waiting time for the new drug approval process.

The author realized that he had deviated too far from the main theme of this article, and this was the place he should stop. He intended to address only fecal transplants and related issues in this article. Unexpectedly, the Ebola epidemic occurred and it attracted the attention of all people, including this author. He has to admit that, unfortunately, now is not the time to address any issues related to the fecal transplant. He felt defeated, just like Betty did. He knows that there are thousands of elders who are suffering from C-diff infections in nursing homes and other elder care facilities. They will not be treated with a quick and easy relief of fecal transplants until they have proven to have recurrent C-diff infections. The consolation is that they do have fecal transplants as the last resource, which was not available only a couple of years ago. Now the author understood Betty's comment about the missed opportunity.

References for Chapter Eleven

* Re. 27: Adams C., Brantner V., "Estimating the cost of the new drug development is really 803 million

dollars?" Health Aff (Millwood) **25** (2); 420-8. (2006)
PMID 16522582

* Ref. 28: History of Federal Regulation: 1962 to
present (on drug and medical devices).
http;//www.fdareview.org/history.shtml

About Yashi Nozawa

Yashi Nozawa was born in Tokyo, Japan. He came to the United States for graduate studies and received M.S and Sc.D. degrees in Aeronautics and Astronautics from MIT. After his retirement from engineering, he began writing as a second career. He writes in two different fields: the genres of biographical fiction and memoirs, and science and religions, specializing in the rational explanation of religious phenomena. He has written several dozen articles in both fields for periodicals. He has also published, "Temporary Permanence", subtitled "My Life in America: Humorous Short Stories Based on Experiences of a Japanese Engineer," a collection of autobiographical short stories. Readers of the book have praised his O. Henry-style writing and made it a local best seller. "Don't Be Afraid of Air Raids" is the second book in his memoir series, but the first book dealing with war experience. It describes his experience in

Doolittle's Tokyo Raid on April 18, 1942 during the earliest part of the Pacific War and its after effects.

In the science-religion series, he published, "The Spring Connections: Easter, Passover, and Others," (as Dr. Yasushi Nozawa). The book is about the deep-rooted tradition of spring celebrations and explains the underlying connection between different religious celebrations in spring time, namely vernal equinox, Passover, and Easter. He also disclosed his new interpretation of the meaning of the Israelites' Exodus from Egypt in the book.

"Betrayal, Resurrection, and Conversion: Three Christian Miracles Explained," is his second book in the science and religion field. He discloses three bold new hypotheses: Three major miracles in Christianity are simple misunderstandings of series of man-made and natural events. He explained how the events happened without evoking the supernatural power of God and without contradicting descriptions in the Bible.

"The First Christmas: A History of Celebration" is his third book in the science-religion series. It covers the origin and evolution of Christmas celebrations and associated events. He wrote in detail about early American exploration, especially the often neglected subject of Christmas celebration among Vikings and other early settlers.